Untwisting the Author's Mind
a 28-day yoga & mediation journey for writers

Mia Michele and
C. Michele Haytko, LD, CBE, CYT, CMT

Infinity House Publishing

Philadelphia

ISBN: 9798356403170

First Printing
2022

Daily Journey

Day 1: Mountain Pose
Day 2: Tree Pose
Day 3: Eagle Pose
Day 4: Downward Dog Pose
Day 5: Bow Pose
Day 6: Thunderbolt Pose
Day 7: Dolphin Pose
Day 8: Butterfly Pose
Day 9: Happy Baby Pose
Day 10: Upward Dog Pose
Day 11: Rabbit Pose
Day 12: Star Pose
Day 13: Horse Pose
Day 14: One-Legged Pigeon Pose
Day 15: Threading the Neele Pose
Day 16: Goddess Pose
Day 17: Pigeon Pose
Day 18: Cobra Pose
Day 19: Boat Pose
Day 20: Triangle Pose
Day 21: Warrior Pose
Day 22: Wheel Pose
Day 23: Child's Pose
Day 24: Dancer Pose
Day 25: Rising Sun Pose
Day 26: Plank Pose
Day 27: Lotus Pose
Day 28: Corpse Pose

I am starting this 28-day journey with the goal of:

____

____

____

Draw, doodle, or place a photo of something that represents how you are feeling right now, at this point in your journey.

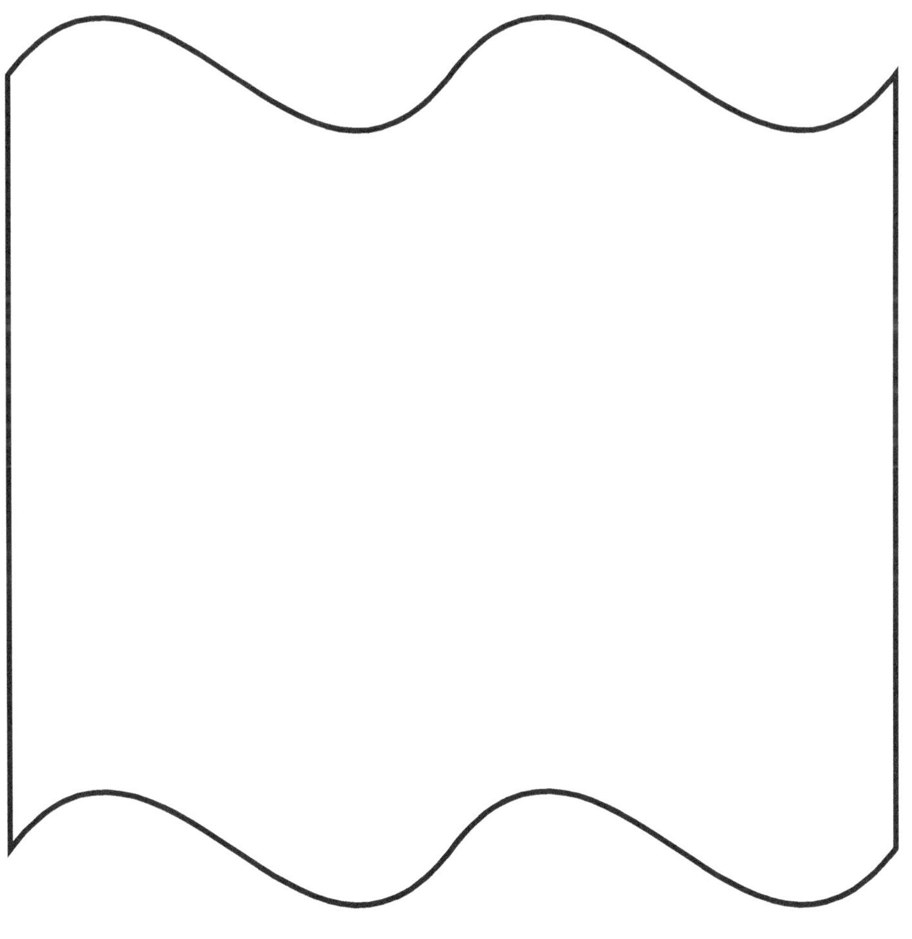

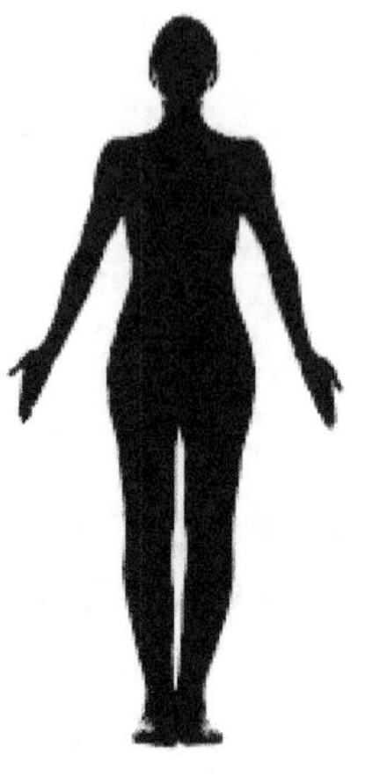

Mountain Pose

Day 1 ~ Date _______________________________

"You are not in the mountains; the mountains are in you."

-John Muir

Stand with your big toes touching. Keep your heels slightly apart and tighten your muscles, feeling a firmness moving through your body. Press your shoulder blades into your back and drop your shoulders, feeling energy moving down your neck and through your spine. Draw your head tall with your chin parallel to the floor. Your arms can be out to your side with your hands open and fingers spread, or you can bring your hands to prayer in front of your chest

Do I feel strong? Do I feel weak? Why? ___________________________

____

____

____

____

____

Strength comes from within, yet at our low points, we cannot reach inside

and find it. Writer's block often creates a sense of weakness. What

situations may be leading to my block? How can I engage my mind and

creative side?

____

____

____

____

____

Day 1

Day 1

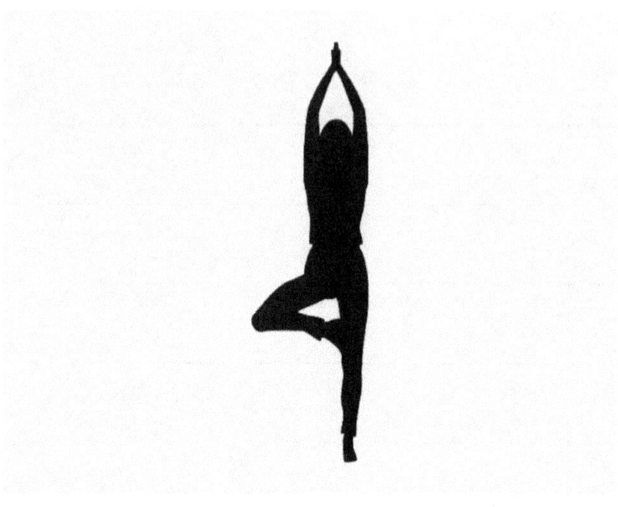

Tree Pose

Day 2 ~ Date _______________________________

"Plants are more courageous than almost all human beings: an orange tree would rather die than produce lemons, whereas instead of dying the average person would rather be someone they are not."
-Mokokoma Mokhonoana

Start in *Mountain* pose for a solid breath. Open your toes and press your feet firmly into the mat. Tighten your abdominals as you breath and gently draw energy down your spine as you lengthen and relax your shoulders downward. As your arms either rise over your head or bend to allow your hands to come into prayer at your chest, raise your right foot high into your left thigh. If this is too difficult, place foot on the shin; do not balance against the knee. Your pelvis should be level, with your hips squared forward. To deepen this posture, you can place your right hand on your heart and take hold of the right foot with your left hand. Focus on your breath and try to take 5 deep breaths here. At completion, return to *Mountain,* and move into the opposite side for a second *Tree* pose.

Am I living authentically? How? Why or why not? _________________

____

____

____

____

Writing for oneself is far more important than success or writing for others.

However, we often have financial (and other) needs to consider that can

hinder our growth as writers. Do you feel like you are forced to live as

someone else? That you are dying inside because you cannot produce your

authentic fruit? ____

____

____

____

____

____

____

Day 2

Day 2

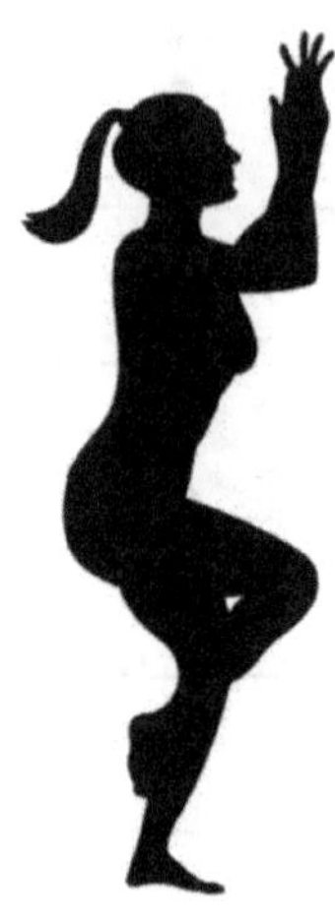

Eagle Pose

Day 3 ~ Date _______________________________

"The eyesight for an eagle is what thought is to a man."
-Dejan Stojanovic

Start in *Mountain* pose and move your feet slightly apart. Lift your arms over your head while pressing your feet into the mat. Reach for the stars while grounding your feet into the earth and lengthen your spine. Bend both knees as you allow your arms to come out to the sides. Lift your right foot and wrap your right thigh over your left before placing your right foot behind your left calf. Slide your arms in front of you and wrap your left arm over your right arm, letting the left elbow cross over the right arm. Bring your right hand to your face as you cross your forearms. Press your hand together in prayer. At completion, return to *Mountain* and move into the opposite side for a second Eagle Pose.

Eagles soar about the clouds and dive in to grab what they want. Do you feel like you are eagle, soaring about and finding what you seek?

____

____

____

____

How can you focus on what you are seeking? What is troubling you? How can you isolate the issues that are keeping you from moving beyond this block and finding your creative streak?

____

____

____

____

____

____

Day 3

Day 3

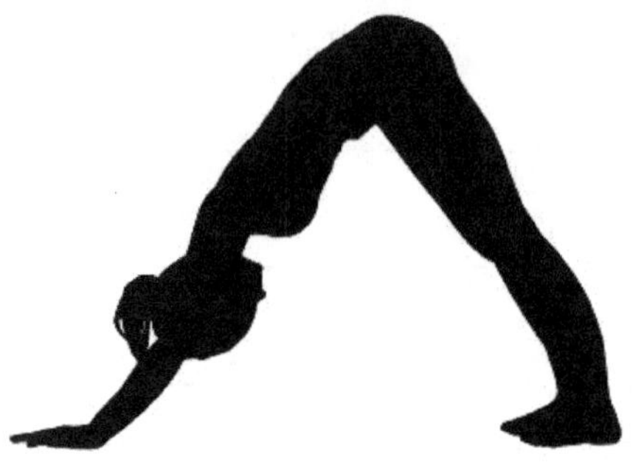

Downward Dog Pose

Day 4 ~ Date _______________________________

"Dogs have boundless enthusiasm but no sense of shame."
-Moby

Start in a *Table* position, on your hands and knees, with your hands in front of your shoulders and your knees directly below your hips. Exhale and lift your knees from the floor. Lengthen your tailbone, lift your sitting bones, and elongate from your ankles through your pelvis. Exhale as you stretch your heels to the floor and straighten your knees. Actively push your hands into the floor as you focus on lengthening your arms. Keep your head between your upper arms and focus on keeping your joints active rather than locked.

Are you still enthusiastic about being a writer? How does writing fuel

you?

____

____

____

____

____

Does writing still feel like a calling and vocation? Or has it devolved into a

job? ____

____

____

____

____

____

____

Day 4

Day 4

17

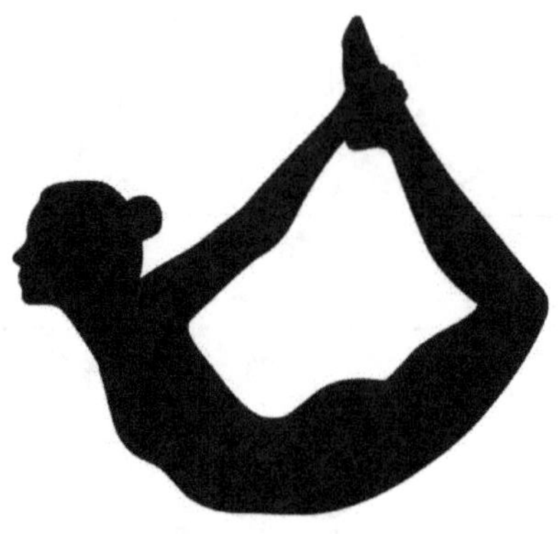

Bow Pose

Day 5 ~ Date _______________________________

"When the archer misses the center of the target, he…seeks for the cause of his failure in himself."
— Confucius

Lie on your belly in *Crocodile* pose. Engage your body, then bend your knees and grab the outer edges of your ankles with your hands. Lift your rib cage and shoulders before lengthening your tailbone. Strengthen and push through your legs as your hands hold onto your ankles as you lift your head to gaze forward, lifting your chest as you press down through your thighs.

The stresses of daily life can ruin our writing practice. They can lead to self-doubt and the fear that our lack of monetary or literary success means that we are wasting our time. They can lead us to misery. What things in your daily life are hindering your writing?

____

____

____

____

Do you feel resentful about your "real life"? How can you work through this? ____

____

____

____

____

____

____

Day 5

Day 5

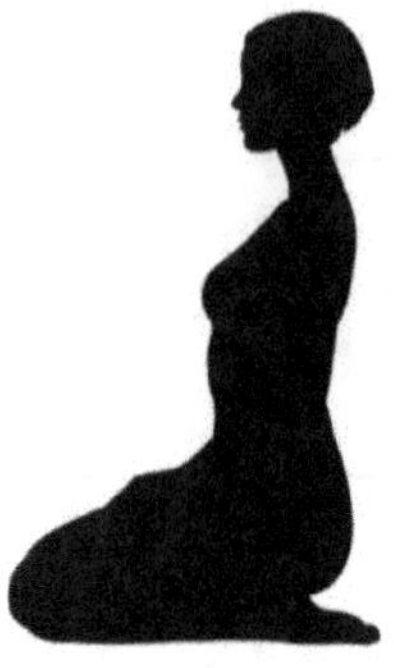

Thunderbolt Pose

Day 6 ~ Date _______________________________

"There are days…when…slow, steady effort is rewarded with justice that arrives like a thunderbolt,"
-Barack Obama

Sit back on your heels with legs bent and your big toes touching. Fold both legs, keeping your hips on the heels. Toes pointing out behind you and big toes touching each other. Keep your head, neck and spine in a straight line with your palms on your thighs and facing up.

Writing is hard work. When writer's block impedes the process, we can often feel like the end product isn't worth our effort. Are you currently in a place of self-rejection? _______________________________________

____

____

____

Could your block be related to your own negative self-image of your talent and worth? ____________________________________

____

____

____

____

____

____

Day 6

Day 6

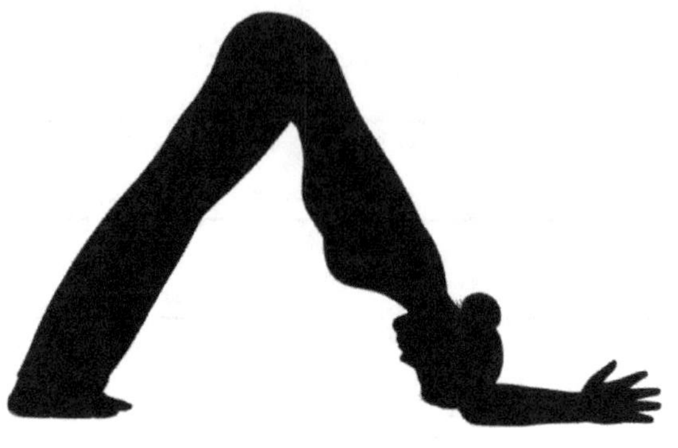

Dolphin Pose

Day 7 ~ Date ______________________________

"In shark infested waters, don't assume the fin coming toward you is a dolphin."
-Mary Russel

Start in a *Table* position, on your hands and knees, with your hands in front of your shoulders and your knees directly below your hips. And move into *Downward Facing Dog* on an exhale, lifting your knees from the floor as you lengthen your tailbone, lift your sitting bones, and elongate from your ankles through your pelvis. Exhale as you stretch your heels to the floor and straighten your knees. Instead of pushing your hands into the floor as you focus on lengthening your arms, drop to your forearms with your hands facing away from you. Keep your head between your upper arms and focus on keeping your joints active rather than locked.

It can be hard to approach writing as a hobby that requires expense rather than an opportunity that creates financial freedom. For some authors, their writing will bring awards and a paycheck that will cover their mortgages (and more!). While some writers will be fortunate enough to have publishing companies that will cover their expenses and agents who will negotiate on their behalf, many writers incur the burden of their travel, conferences, and publications on their own. It can be easy to trust those who look like they want to help- only to be burned in the in. The fear of this as well as the stress of falling for fraudulent assistance can create emotional hurdles to overcome. Are you in a position such as this? Could this be negatively impacting your writing headspace?

____

____

____

____

____

____

Day 7

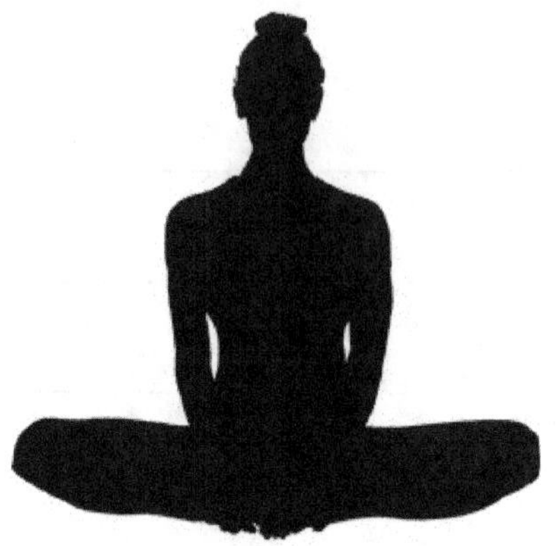

Butterfly Pose

"Wings are of many kinds. Butterfly's wings,...dragonfly's serene wings,...lovely wings of humming birds, tiny wings of a fly or a bumble-bee...[and] they fly their best according to their ability of flying. We should not underestimate the size of those heavenly wings."
-Munia Khan

Sit with your spine straight and join the soles of your feet by bending your knees. Pull your lower body in as far toward your pelvis as is comfortable. Hold both your feet tightly with your hands. As you breathe deeply, press the thighs and knees down towards the floor. To deepen the pose, length your back and lay your torso over your bent legs. After a few deep breaths, return to an upright position.

It is so easy to compare ourselves to others. Even when we appreciate the

success of others, it is hard to not look at their news- amazing presales,

bestseller numbers, significant royalties- and compare. That can lead to

negative self-image and an inability to encourage. Have you been

comparing recently? How could this be impacting your ability to write

and create? ____

____

____

____

____

____

____

____

____

____

Day 8

Day 8

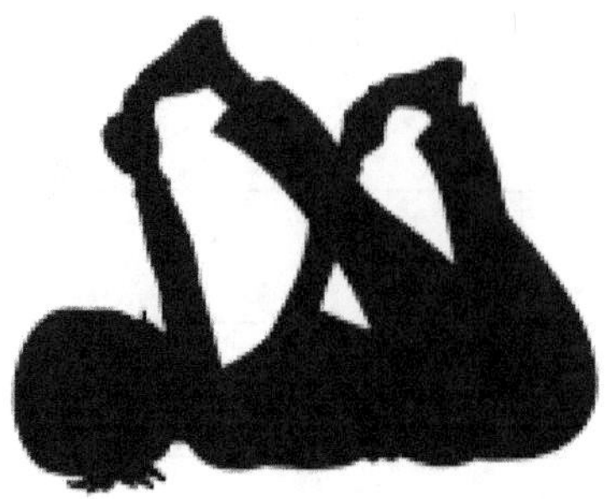

Happy Baby Pose

Day 9 ~ Date _______________________________

"The moment a child is born, the mother is also born."
-Bhagwan Shree Rajneesh

Lie on your back and bend your knees into your belly. On an inhale, grip the outsides of your feet with your hands, bending your knees if needed. Open your knees slightly wider than your torso, then bring them up toward your armpits. Position each ankle directly over the knee, so your shins are perpendicular to the floor. Alternate an easy pressure on your feet as you pull and lengthen them, rolling gently on the floor as desired.

Am I a real writer? Who among us has not asked that question, tainted with our own fears of the answer? Our projects, like children, are birthed from us, a conception of idea and image crafted into words through the artful act of writing. At the writing of the first word, we are writers, something new birthed from the chaos before. Are you struggling with your writer identity? Are you self-impeding by not owning who you truly are?

Day 9

Day 9

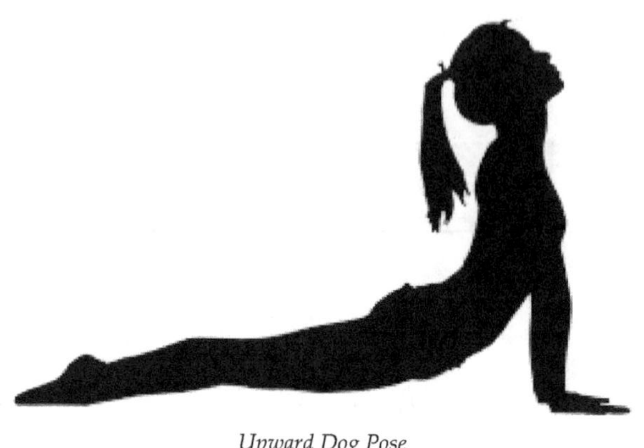

Upward Dog Pose

Day 10 ~ Date _______________________________

"We come to the page with too many expectations… We don't just want a good book; we want a bestseller. If it isn't perfect, we hate it. If it isn't 100% right, it's 1000% wrong… It's all or nothing with us and that's the kind of dichotomy that shanks our happiness… So: care less. Ease off the stress stick. Have more fun with what you're doing. When your kids and dogs play in the mud, you can either freak out that they're too dirty, or you can laugh and jump in the mud, too…. Jump in the…mud already."
- Chuck Wendig

Lower your body into a *Plank* position. As your body approaches the ground, inhale to straighten your arms as you roll your toes under the tops of your feet. Don't bring your thighs to the floor. Open your chest toward the ceiling as you straighten your arms, but don't drop your head back. Keep your legs engaged and drop your hips toward the floor. Push strongly into the palms and toes. Keep your shoulders over your wrists and draw your shoulder blades down and toward your spine to create space between your shoulders and your ears.

What expectations have you placed on yourself as a writer? Am you

writing   for   yourself?   For   others?   For   success?

____

____

____

____

What kind of stress comes each time you open a file or look at a blank

page? Are you losing yourself to find fame and money? Are you waiting

to publish because nothing is perfect? How much stress is your dream

putting on you because of your expectations and desires?

____

____

____

____

____

____

Day 10

41

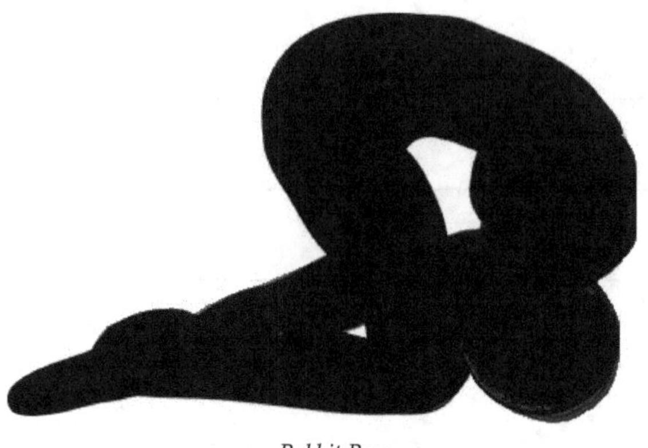

Rabbit Pose

Day 11 ~ Date _______________________

"Ideas are like rabbits. You get a couple and learn how to handle them, and pretty soon you have a dozen."
-John Steinbeck

From *Child* pose, hold onto the heels with the hands and pull the forehead in towards the knees with the top of the head on the floor. Inhale and lift the hips up towards the ceiling as you roll onto your crown, pressing your forehead close to your knees.

How many of us have file after file of idea on our computer? It seems that, as soon as we have one great story idea, another pops in... And then another... And another! Focus can be so difficult to achieve when we have so many *great ideas* living in our heads. Is there a story you are desperate to work on, but another idea supersedes your progress? What issue might you be running from (and running to a new idea) that stops you from working on the piece that you feel called to complete? _______

____

____

____

____

____

____

____

____

____

Day 11

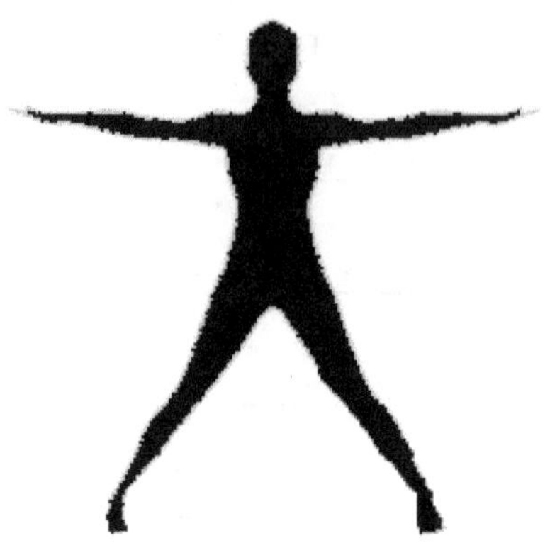

Star Pose

Day 12 ~ Date _______________________

"Without the dark, we'd never see the stars."
- Stephenie Meyer

Begin in *Mountain* pose and rest your hands on your hips. Step your feet wide apart and turn your toes to the corners of your mat. Extend your arms out to the sides at shoulder-height with your palms facing forward. Press down through your heels and straighten your legs. Inhale as you elongate through your torso. Exhale and release your shoulder blades away from your head, toward the back of your waist. Spread your fingers and reach out strongly through your fingertips.

Self-doubt is like a cancer. It starts small and then grows until it takes over everything. But in our darkest days, we can find the spark of creativity that encourages us to keep dreaming, to keep going, to write one more word. What is your greatest doubt? What is impeding you from seeing your star shine brightly? ______________________________

____

____

____

____

____

____

____

____

____

Day 12

Day 12

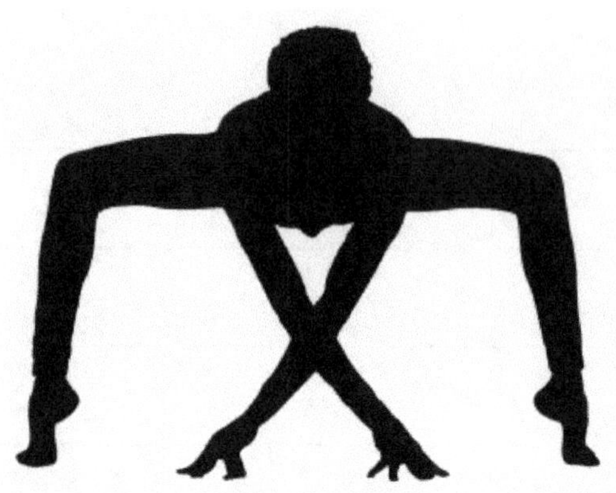

Horse Pose

Day 13 ~ Date _______________________________

"A horse who bears himself proudly is a thing of such beauty and astonishment that he attracts the eyes of all beholders."
-Xenophon

From a standing position step feet apart slightly wider than shoulder-distance, toes pointing outward. As you inhale reach arms overhead wide pressing palms together. As you exhale bend knees 90 degrees and pull hands to chest sliding your shoulder blades downward. Slowly slide your hands to the floor, crossing the arms and pressing the fingertips into the mat. Keep your back straight and your gaze forward.

We live in a time of keyboard warriors who leave bad reviews and insult writers instead of giving constructive criticism that allows an artist to flourish and grow. It can be all too easy to sink down and insult people in return when they attack the work of our souls. Holding ourselves to a higher esteem can be difficult but will always prove right. Are you struggling with the harsh words of another? How can you turn that negativity into self-growth? _________________________________

____

____

____

____

____

____

____

____

Day 13

Day 13

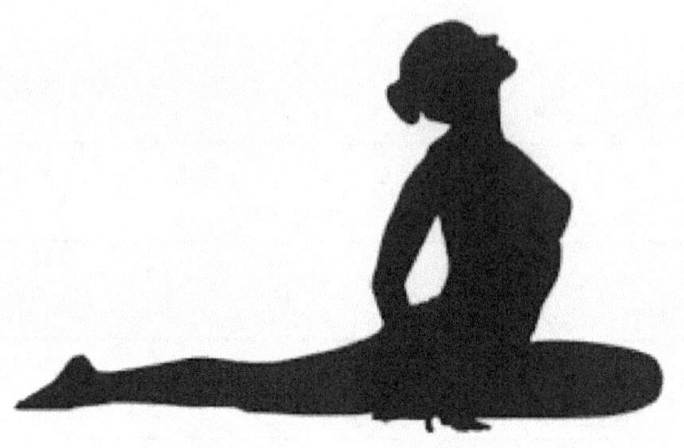

One-Legged Pigeon Pose

Day 14 ~ Date _______________________________

"Sometimes you are the pigeon, and sometimes you are the statue."
-Claude Chabrol

Starting in *Table* pose, slide your left knee forward, angling your left shin under your torso so your left foot is at the front of your right knee and the outside of your left shin is resting on the floor. Slowly slide your right leg back, straightening your knee and resting the top of your thigh on the floor. Lower your outer left backside to the floor and position your left heel just in front of your right hip. Lift your torso away from your thigh. Lengthen your lower back by pressing your tailbone down and forward. To deepen the pose, release your hands one by one, and lower your torso over the left leg and down to the floor, keeping the spine long and resting the forehead on the floor or your forearms. Come up with an inhale and return to your hands and knees to repeat on the other side.

Sometimes reviews are great; sometimes they are horrific. It is easy to read the good ones and let them drift away while internalizing the negative ones. Both are useful for growth and future creativity.

What is your favorite positive review? How does it make you a better writer in the future? _______________________________________

____

____

____

____

What is your least-favorite negative review? How can you transform it into constructive criticism? _______________________________

____

____

____

____

____

Day 14

Day 14

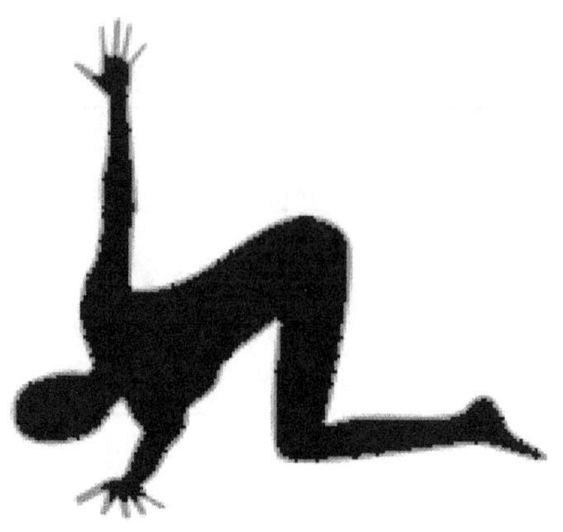

Threading the Neele Pose

Day 15 ~ Date _______________________________

"Between threading a needle and raving insanity is the smallest eye in creation."
- Caitlin Thomas

Begin in *Table* pose. Slide your left arm forward and extend your right arm out to your side. Thread your right arm under your left arm until your right shoulder and ear are on the mat. To deepen the pose, lift your left arm to the sky. Plant your left hand in front of your face and press back into *Table* position. Repeat on the other side.

Writer's block... The nightmare and bane of every author's existence. Writing is like breathing; when you can't do it, you feel like you are dying. Are you struggling with a next scene, new character, first book? Is there an idea that you cannot grasp, that feels just slightly out of reach? The creative spark is a tiny flicker that grows into a flame. Grab hold of the spark and free write it until it becomes what you are looking for.

Day 15

Day 15

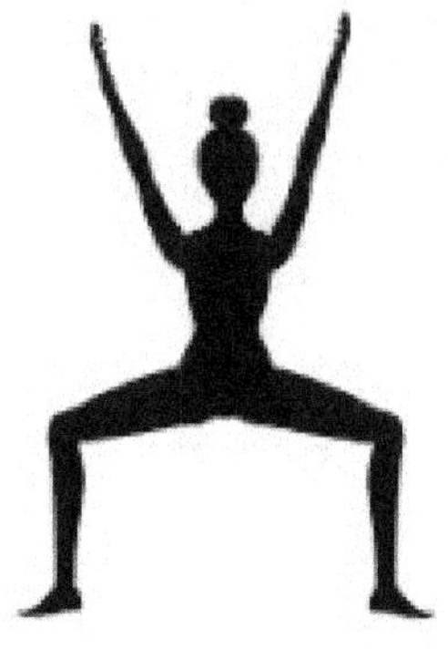

Goddess Pose

Day 16 ~ Date _______________________________

"The Goddess falls in love with Herself, drawing forth her own emanation, which takes on a life of its own. Love of self for self is the creative force of the universe."
- Starhawk

Start in a wide standing stance. Turn your toes out and your heels in, so your feet are pointed out at about a 45-degree angle. Bend your knees and lower your hips down, creating dual 90-degree angles. Reach your arms out and bend your elbows so that your fingertips point skyward. Spread your fingertips wide and activate the muscles across your back. Engage your core muscles and draw your tailbone toward the floor while keeping your spine elongated.

Loving ourselves is a fundamental root of our writing tree. Do you love

yourself? Are you in love with who you are? Why or why not? ________

____

____

____

____

____

How can you better love yourself? How can you create and mold yourself

into a person you would be in love with? How can you find your creative

goddess   (or   god)   within?   ____________________________

____

____

____

____

Day 16

Day 16

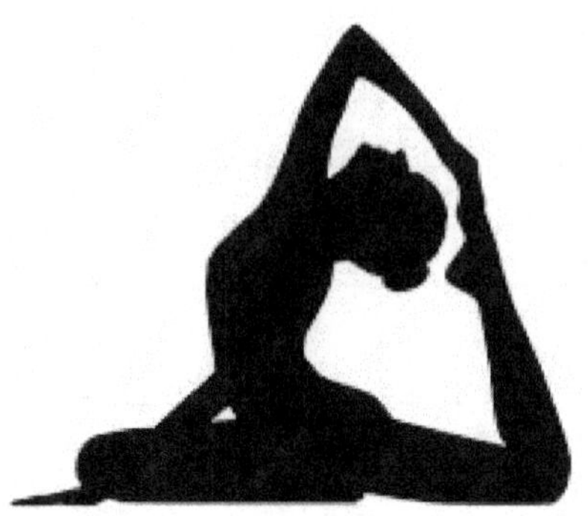

Pigeon Pose

Day 17 ~ Date _______________________________

If the pigeon house does not lack food, it will not lack pigeons; good hope is better than a bad holding."
-Miguel De Cervantes Saavedra

Starting in *Table* pose, slide into *One-Legged Pigeon* pose by moving your left knee forward and angling your left shin under your torso so your left foot is at the front of your right knee and the outside of your left shin is resting on the floor. Slowly slide your right leg back, straightening your knee and resting the top of your thigh on the floor. Lower your outer left backside to the floor and position your left heel just in front of your right hip. Lift your torso away from your thigh. Lengthen your lower back by pressing your tailbone down and forward. Bend your right leg as you reach behind you with your left hand to touch the right toes. Release your foot and lower your leg on an inhale, returning to your hands and knees to repeat on the other side.

You cannot write without ideas. While we often joke about *work in progress* piles, the truth is we need those WIP files. We need the constant influx of ideas, even if they never flesh out into stories or novels. What are some ideas that you currently have floating around? Use those ideas (whether you write them into books or not) to be fuel for your passion.

Day 17

Day 17

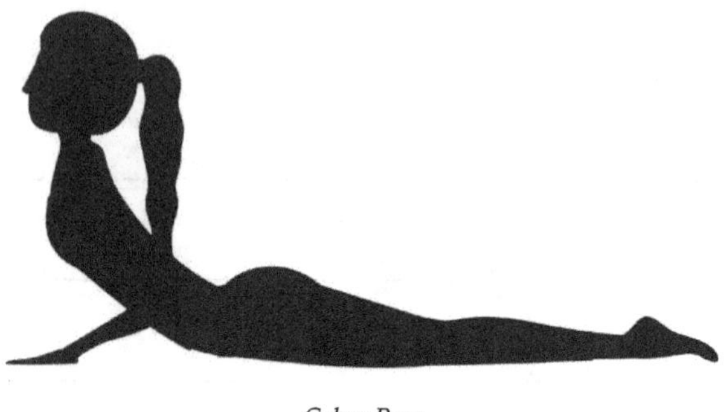

Cobra Pose

Day 18 ~ Date _______________________________

"Fiction [is] like goading a mongoose and a cobra into battle and staying with them to see who wins."
- Shauna Singh Baldwin

Lay on your belly with your feet hip-distance apart and your hands beside your ribs. Pressing down lightly with your hands, lift your head and chest. Roll your shoulders back and down. Keep the back of your neck long and lift your sternum. Straighten your arms while keeping your shoulders away from your ears with a slight bend in your elbows.

Often when I'm writing, I feel the struggle between the selfish nature of the artist and the selfless nature of the mother. My family needs me to be present, but when I'm in *the zone*, I can't be present to anything or anyone but the voices in my head. Life is full of both good and bad; as Swami Satchidananda states: "There is not good without bad...Even Cobra poison can be used as medicine." At its core, I believe artistry is part of the good. However, it can lead us to neglect other things in our lives. Are there things you are neglecting? How can you help your selfish and selfless natures coexist? _________________________________

____

____

____

____

____

____

____

____

Day 18

Day 18

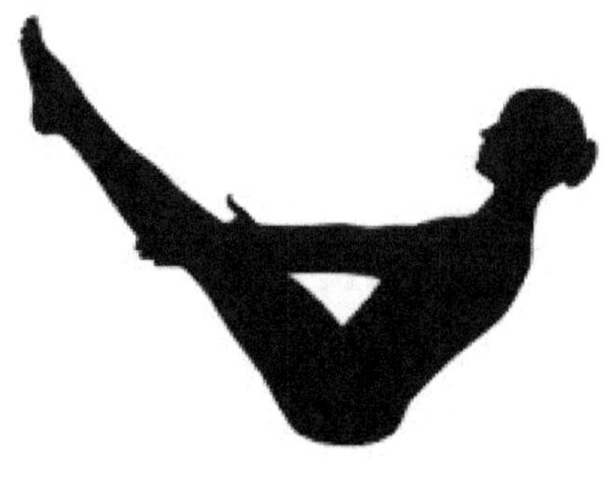

Boat Pose

Day 19 ~ Date _______________________________

"Boats in the harbor are safe but that is not what they are meant for."
- Zig Ziglar

Sit on the floor with your legs straight in front of you. Press your hands on the floor a little behind your hips. Lift through the top of the sternum and lean back slightly. Balance your weight on your sitting bones and tailbone. Exhale and bend your knees, then lift your thighs so they are angled in a 45-degree angle. Slowly straighten your knees. Draw your shoulders back and extend both arms parallel to the floor, with your palms facing in. Point your toes or flex through your heels.

Are you a published author? ____

Publishing is much like birthing a child. It grows within you and then is

there for the world to see, to comment on, to judge. It can be terrifying.

Judgement sits in all sorts of places. Are you a published writer? Do you

have an agent? Are you published by a large publisher? Do you publish

with a small publishing house? Are you independently published? Every

question comes with a hidden (or, at times, not-so-hidden) judgement.

What is holding you into the safe zone of sharing your work with the

world? What struggles are you facing that keep you "in the harbor"?

____

____

____

____

____

____

____

____

Day 19

Day 19

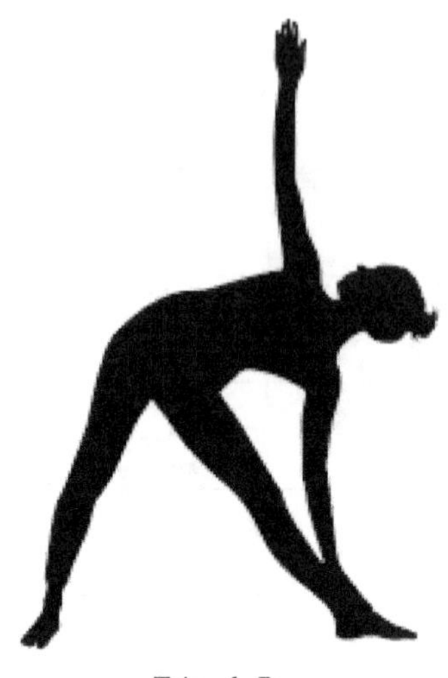

Triangle Pose

Day 20 ~ Date _______________________________

"Love is made up of three unconditional properties in equal measure: acceptance, understanding, and appreciation. Remove any one…and the triangle falls apart."
- Vera Nazarian

From *Mountain* pose, step your feet 3-feet apart. Raise your arms parallel to the floor and reach to the sides. Turn your left foot in slightly and your right foot out to 90 degrees. Firm your thighs and rotate your right thigh outward. Exhale and extend your torso to the right, bending from your hip joint. Reach over the plane of the right leg as you anchor your left hip and press the left heel into the floor. Hinge at the hip and bring the torso to the right, moving your upper body parallel to the floor. Reach your right hand down toward the floor and stretch your left arm toward the ceiling. Open your torso to the left, keeping the left and right sides of the torso equally long. Let the left hip come slightly forward and lengthen the tailbone toward the back heel. Rest your right hand on your right foot, and keep your head in a neutral position, turning to look up at your hand or down at the ground.

Vera Nazarian writes that love is comprised of acceptance, understanding, and appreciation. To love ourselves, we need to embrace acceptance of who we are, understanding of how our minds work, and appreciation for our uniqueness and diversity. How can you encourage and live a life of acceptance, understanding, and appreciation for yourself?

____

____

____

____

____

____

____

____

____

Day 20

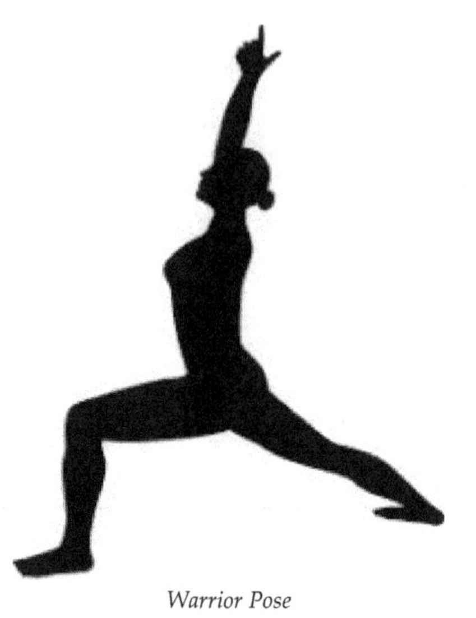

Warrior Pose

Day 21 ~ Date _______________________

"A warrior's greatest glory is not in never falling, but in rising every time we fall."
- Confucius

From *Downward Dog* pose, step your right foot forward so your toes are in line with your fingertips, and shift your foot slightly to the right as you bend your front knee into a 90-degree angle. Pivot your left heel to the floor so your foot forms a 45-degree angle to the side of the mat. Raise your torso and reach your arms up. Open your shoulder blades and bring your palms together and look up at your thumbs.

There will be great stories that fade into the abyss, and there will be lousy stories that hook the public to become bestsellers. Even books with high critical acclaim often do not find commercial success. But when you are the author of a *great story* and cannot understand why books poorly written or without creativity are flying high while you are scraping to get readers, it can be a huge hit to not only your pocketbook but your writer-ego as well. It can make you want to stop writing altogether. Are you finding it hard to rise and write again after poor reviews or positive reviews with poor sales? How can you train yourself to be a warrior writer instead of a worrier writer? ___________________

____

____

____

____

____

____

____

Day 21

Day 21

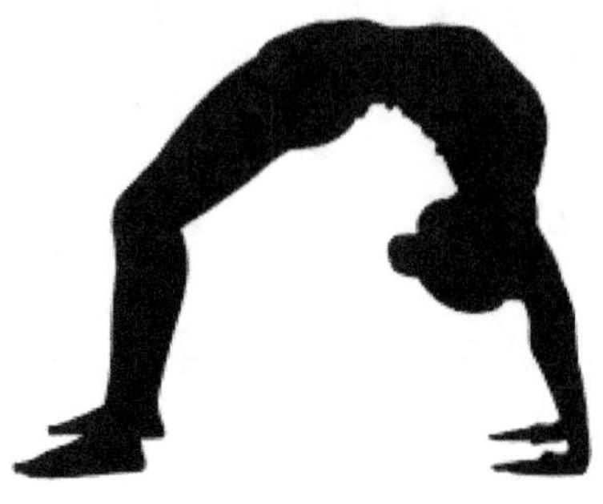

Day 22 ~ Date _______________________________

"Get up and set your shoulder to the wheel...As you have come into this world, leave some mark behind."
- Swami Vivekananda

Lie on your back, with your knees bent, and walk your feet close to your bottom as you reach your fingertips toward your heels. The feet should be parallel and hips' distance apart. Bend your elbows and move your hands to beneath your shoulders with your fingers pointed at your feet. Inhale and press into your hands and your feet as you lift off the floor. Keep your elbows and feet parallel, and do not apply pressure to the neck while your head still rests on the floor. Straighten your arms as you lift your head off the floor, opening your chest as you rise and elongating through the body as your legs straighten into the full *Wheel* pose.

We are all desperate to write the scenes and voices in our heads. That is the writing that is for us. But then we feel the need to leave something of ourselves behind, some piece of us that will show our life was full- that we made a mark on the world. What is your goal for yourself? Are you content with making a mark within your own world, or do you feel the need to pursue public success in order to leave your mark on the world at large? ____

____

____

____

____

____

____

____

____

____

Day 22

Day 22

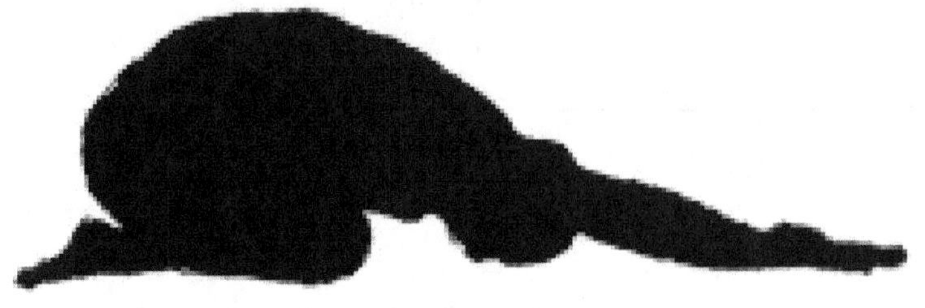

Child's Pose

Day 23 ~ Date _______________________________

"The final stage of wisdom is becoming a kid again."
- Maxime Lagacé

Move into a *Table* pose, coming onto your hands and knees. Spread your knees, keeping the tops of your feet on the floor with the big toes touching, as you bring your belly to the ground, shifting your weight to deep between your thighs and resting your forehead on the floor. Relax your body as you breathe deeply into the pose.

Oh, to be a child! To believe that nothing is impossible, that we can start again anew tomorrow, that words (and negative reviews) cannot hurt us. Children have an innocence that hasn't been buried beneath experience and introspection. Have you lost your inner child? Are you struggling to write through your thoughts so that you can find the story within? How can you embrace the true wisdom of returning to a childhood mind?

Day 23

Day 23

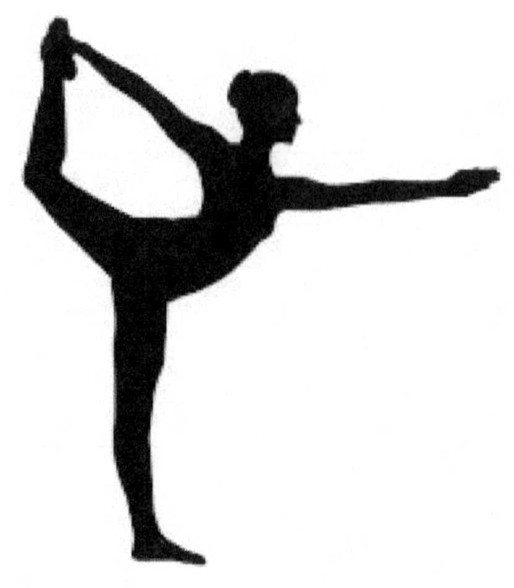

Dancer Pose

Day 24 ~ Date ______________________________

"We dance for laughter, we dance for tears, we dance for madness, we dance for fears, we dance for hopes, we dance for screams, we are the dancers, we create the dreams."
-Albert Einstein

Start in *Mountain* pose. Shift your weight into your right foot and slowly lift your left heel towards your left butt cheek. Catch the inner arch of your left foot with your left hand and find your balance. Extend your right arm forward (while keeping it parallel to the floor) and lower your chest forward as you raise the left knee. Press the top of your left foot into your hand, lifting your left heel away from your bottom. Reverse the position to return to *Mountain* pose and repeat on the other side.

Writing is a symphony through reality, fantasy, and every space between! Sometimes, we are the dancer- floating through the music on a dream, writing the stories and people from our thoughts. Other times, we are the dance, suffering through writer's block, angsty at perceived perception of our labors, crying along with the sorrows and laughing with the joys of our characters. Where are you currently in this masterpiece? Are you the dancer or the dance at present? ____________

____

____

____

____

____

____

____

____

____

Day 24

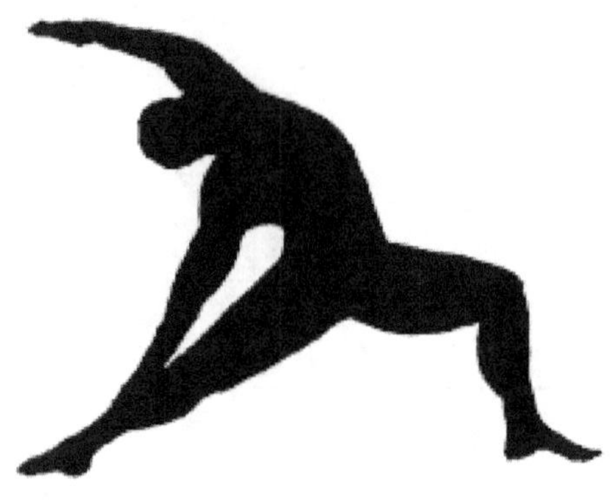

Rising Sun Pose
(aka Sun Warrior Pose)

Day 25 ~ Date _______________________________

"Every sunrise is a new chapter...waiting to be written."
- Juansen Dizon

Come into a *Warrior* pose by first stepping your right foot forward so your toes are in line with your fingertips and shifting your foot slightly to the right as you bend your front knee into a 90-degree angle. Pivot your left heel to the floor so your foot forms a 45-degree angle to the side of the mat. Raise your torso and reach your arms up. Open your shoulder blades and bring your palms together and look up at your thumbs. Deepen into *Rising Sun* by lifting your right hand up to the ceiling while shifting your week into a lunge as you lengthen through your left leg. Drop your left hand back to your left ankle and look to the sky at your raised right hand as it arcs over the body.

On days where we try to write and nothing happens, we can almost convince ourselves to give up. But tomorrow is a new day. Today's writer's block is tomorrow's climax. It is always darkest before the sunrise, and day wouldn't be as welcomed if not for the night before it. Pick up the pen, abide with the night, and work through into the sunrise. What are you struggling to put into words right now? _______________

____

____

____

____

____

____

____

____

____

Day 25

Day 25

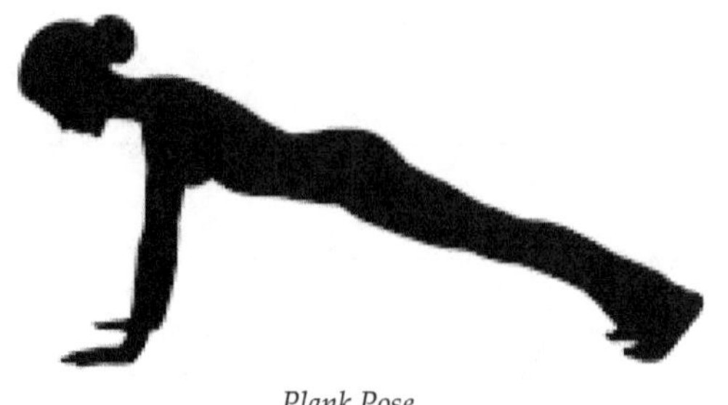

Plank Pose

Day 26 ~ Date _______________________________

"They [who] do not appreciate to the full a clear sky...have never entrusted their lives to the mercy of four planks on a raging sea."
- Alexandre Dumas

Begin in *Table* pose, on your hands and knees, with your hands under your shoulders and your knees under your hips. Spread your fingers wide on the mat and center your balance. One at a time, straighten your legs behind you, pressing into the balls of your feet. Engage your legs as you lift, drawing your belly button into your spine and tightening your core as you settle into a traditional push-up position.

Henry David Thoreau.   Emily Dickinson. John Kennedy Toole. Kate Chopin. John Keats. Edgar Allan Poe. Franz Kafka. Sylvia Plath. What do these writers all have in common? They were relatively unknown during their lives. How much do you think they would have appreciated knowing that one day their work would be loved and revered? Although you may never find commercial success in your lifetime, write with the knowledge that you never know what might be held in tomorrow. Appreciate the idea, even if you never see it come to pass. Is this something you think you can do? Do you have thoughts about what your success might look like one day? Will it be all the sweeter because of your struggle to get there? ___________________

____

____

____

____

____

____

Day 26

Day 26

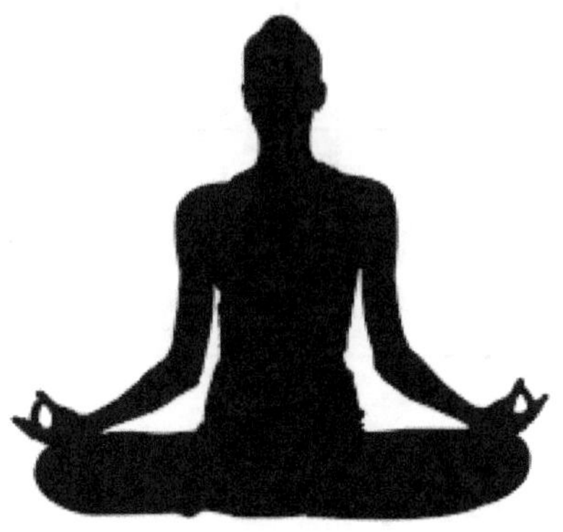

Lotus Pose

Day 27 ~ Date _______________________________

"Just like the lotus we too have the ability to rise from the mud, bloom out of the darkness, and radiate into the world."
- Unknown

Sit on the floor with your legs extended. Bend your right knee and cradle your knee and your foot in your hands. Rotate your leg from the hip- not the knee- and guide your foot into your left hip crease. Repeat this on the opposite side as you bend your left knee and cradle your knee and your foot in your hands before rotating your leg from the hip, lifting your shin to guide the left foot over the right, and tucking it into the right hip crease. Settle the tops of your feet against your upper thighs and release your knees toward the floor. Sit up tall, lifting your sternum as you lengthen your spine while taking slow, deep breaths.

Do you feel like writing has been an easy journey for you? When did you

know you wanted to be a writer? How long have you been writing?

____

____

____

____

A cut flower is beautiful, but it will wither no matter how much attention

you offer it. That which grows will eventually die but will be born again.

Do you feel like you are a root underground or that you have been born

from the soil? Are you writing as though you are in bloom or like you

have been cut? _______________________________________

____

____

____

____

Day 27

108

Day 27

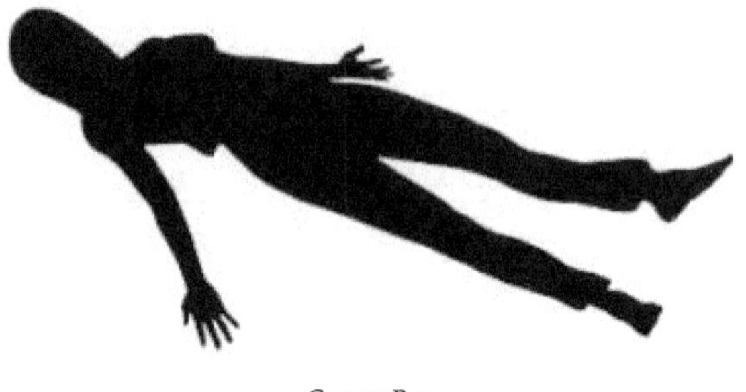

Corpse Pose

Day 28 ~ Date _______________________________

"Writing is a deeper sleep than death. Just as one wouldn't pull a corpse from its grave, I can't be dragged from my desk at night."
-Franz Kafka

Often called the most difficult posture to achieve, *Corpse* pose is a perfect way to end each practice. Lie down on your back. Relax and separate your legs, letting your feet can fall open to either side. Bring your arms alongside your body and turn your palms up, relaxing the hands and fingers. One section as a time, begin to relax your whole body, feeling heavy and sinking into the floor into the floor as you breathe deeply. Starting at either the top or bottom of the body, release the stress and tension from each section: head, neck, and face; shoulders, arms, hands, and fingers; torso and back; abdominals and pelvis; hips and legs; and the feet and toes. Breathe deeply but normally, focusing on the breath as you release tension and move into a meditative state.

Stephen King once said, "Talent is cheaper than table salt. What separates the talented individual from the successful one is a lot of hard work." When we are fueled by creativity and trapped at our computers by the voices in our minds, we put our very souls down on paper. But sometimes the talented voice just isn't enough to bring the greatest novel to life for others. And that's okay. We have to be content writing for ourselves and deciding whether or not we want to work at success. Being a writer is as easy as breathing. Being a successful author requires a lot of sacrifice and hardship. Where are you on your journey? Are you in love with writing so that no word is a missed opportunity? Are you tired from book tours, conventions, and solicitations? Are you inspired by book signings and speaking on panels? Are you writing for your eyes alone? Embrace the journey and what you want from it. Don't hold yourself to the lofty ideals and dreams of others. Go bravely in the direction that you wish to walk.

____

____

____

Day 28

I ended this 28-day journey by:

____

____

____

Draw, doodle, or place a photo of something that represents how you are feeling right now, at this point in your journey.

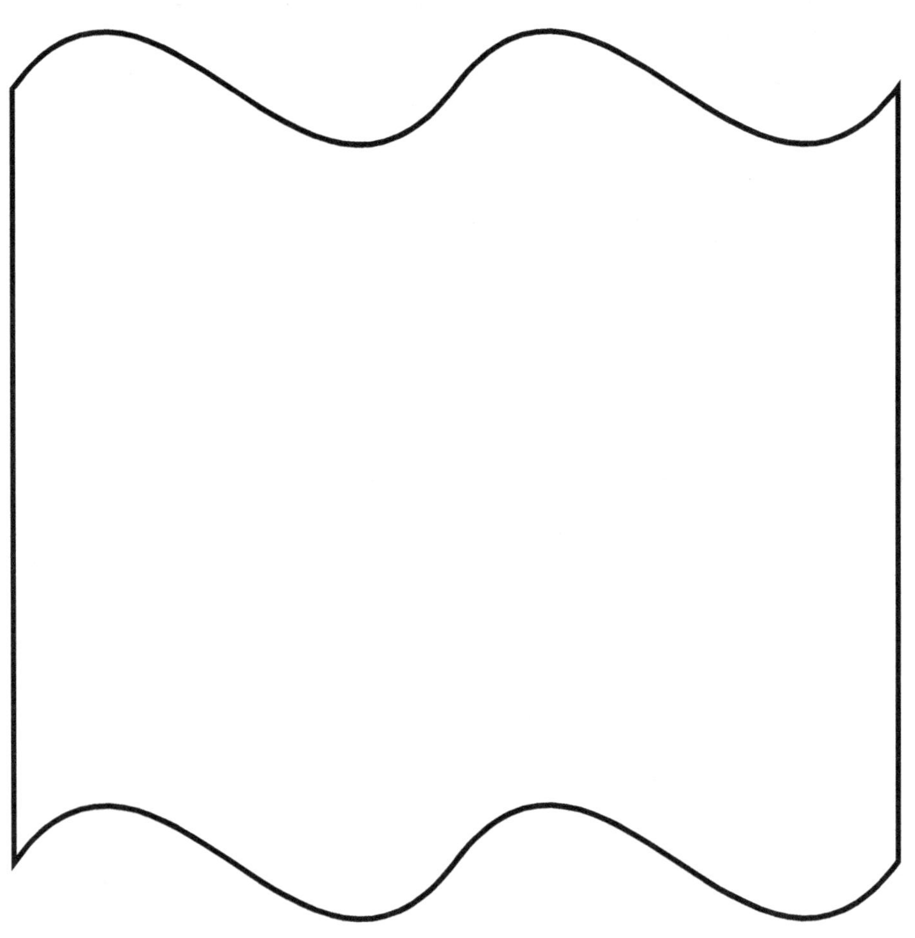

About the Authors

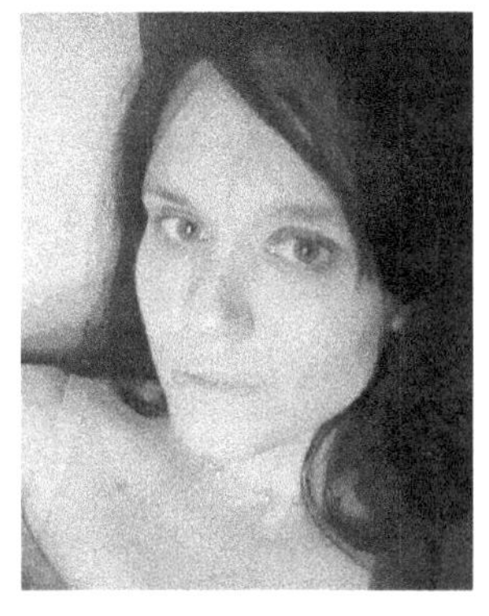

Mia Michele is the author of multiple romance novels, including the bestselling Mafia romance, <u>Faultline</u>, the dystopian <u>Vale</u>, and her most recent, a retelling of the Persephone-Hades myth, <u>The Gospel of Persephone</u>. She can often be found drinking too much coffee in local Pennsylvania coffee shops or lecturing on BDSM and romance culture. A mother of a gaggle of children, she spends way too little time running and too much time keeping her house clean. She often brings her muse (and husband) with her to conferences, where he can sometimes be found lurking in presentations or fueling her coffee addiction. Visit her online at www.miamichele.com.

C. Michele Haytko, LD, CBE, CYT, CMT, was trained as a labor doula and childbirth educator by Birth Arts International and was certified to teach mediation and yoga through Aura Yoga, with additional certifications for prenatal & postnatal yoga. She specializes in bereavement work and has served dozens in the PA-NY-NJ-MD area. Her service organization, Mending Heart Bellies, utilizes therapeutic talk sessions to 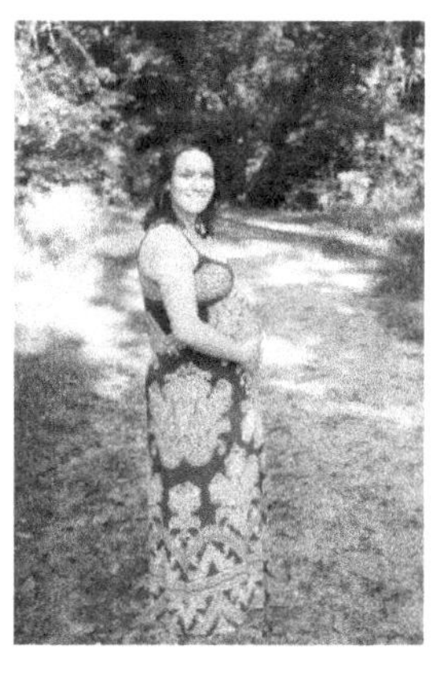 help those suffering from loss and grief, navigating affair recovery and eating disorders, and understanding themselves. Visit her online or find a list of her publications at www.mendingheartbellies.org.

Find your next book at www.miamichele.com

<u>Fiction by Mia Michele:</u>

Amnesty of the Heart (Aegean Affairs, #1)

Drunk on Passion (Aegean Affairs, #2)

Happily Ever After (Aegean Affairs, #3)

Aegean Affairs Duet #1

Martial Hearts (The Club, #1)

Hosts and Hellions: the complete trilogy

Children of Hellions (Hosts and Hellions, #1)

Sons of God (Hosts and Hellions, #2)

Daughters of Men (Hosts and Hellions, #3)

Vale

Faultline

The Gospel of Persephone

Untwisting the Author's Mind